Hormones Gone Wild
A Men's Survival Guide
to Menopause Mayhem

WARNING!
Approach With Caution, Chocolate and a Fan

Ella Morgan

Copyright Pickle & Pen Press 2024

So, here you are, flipping through this book, likely with a mix of curiosity and a desperate hope that it holds the key to surviving... well, let's just call it Menopausal Madness.

Congratulations, my friend, you're officially in the thick of it: the wild, unpredictable, and occasionally downright scary world of menopause. You're about to experience a phase that will test your patience, push your limits, and, at times, make you question your sanity. If you're holding this book, take a deep breath and know you're not alone.

Let's get this straight right off the bat: menopause is no joke. For the women experiencing it, it's a full-blown biological rollercoaster that affects everything from body temperature to emotions - and yes, even the seemingly innocent things you say or do.

Hot flashes, sleepless nights, and mood swings that could rival a thunderstorm are just the tip of the iceberg. Menopause is frustrating, exhausting, and sometimes even downright miserable for her.

So while this book is packed with humor and (hopefully) some survival tips to keep you out of the doghouse, let's take a moment to recognize what she's dealing with: an intense, life altering transition that isn't easy for anyone.

In these pages, you'll find everything from mood trackers to hot flash survival strategies, complete with the kind of humor that'll keep you laughing even when you're dodging side eyes and hiding behind a fan.

The laughs are here to help you both get through it, not to trivialize her experience. With a little patience, empathy, and the ability to find humor in the chaos, you might just come out on the other side a little wiser - and maybe even with a few good stories to tell.

So grab a pen, maybe a bar of chocolate (for her and for you), and let's get you ready to navigate the heat waves, emotional detours, and surprise mood swings ahead.

Buckle up - it's going to be one hell of a ride. But you've got this. And she's got you. Together, you'll make it through, with a bit of snark, a lot of chocolate, and maybe an ice pack or two.

Ella Morgan

Finding your way around
A Men's Survial Guide to Menopause

- It could be a good idea to memorise it for quick reference

The Menopausal Weather Forecast 6

Hot Flash Readiness Kit 10

Mood Swing Bingo 13

Snack Pacification Handbook 16

Man Cave Escape Plan 19

The Pillow Fort Refuge 22

The Menopause First Aid Kit 26

Menopause Proof Conversation Guide 30

The Eye-Roll Counter 34

Chill Level Tracker 37

Sage Advice You Wish You Hadn't Given 41

The Apology Bingo 45

The Side Eye Diary 49

The Temperature of the Room 52

Chocolate Bribery Log 56

Moods to Dodge Today 60

The "Can I Help?" Gauge 64

End-of-the-Day Debrief 69

The "Keep Your Mouth Shut" Game 72

The Menopausal Mood Dictionary 76

Top 10 Things You Should Never, Ever Say 80

Weekly Survival Scorecard 84

Future Planning: The Survival Kit Restock Guide 88

25 Menopause Survival Multiple Choice Quiz 92

Daily Survival Prompts - Mini 30 Day Journal 104

Final Thoughts 114

The Menopausal Weather Forecast

Introduction
If you thought mood swings were intense before, you're in for a wild ride. Think of this as your Menopausal Weather Forecast, because every day is its own damn adventure. The forecast will help you navigate through sunshine, thunderstorms, or a full-on Category 5 hurricane of emotions.

You'll need this guide if you're going to make it through unscathed, or at least with most of your sanity. So, buckle up and check today's forecast before you put your foot in your mouth. Let's see what kind of mood you're up against.

Today's Forecast Tracker
Circle today's mood prediction and prepare your survival strategy accordingly:

Sunny
The stars have aligned! She's feeling good, the world is bright, and it's safe to joke around. Take advantage of this rare moment and plan something fun. Hell, you might even get to use the TV remote tonight.

Partly Cloudy
Approach with caution. She's in a neutral mood but could swing either way. Keep the conversation light and the snacks nearby. She's not quite stormy, but don't press your luck.

Overcast
There's tension in the air, my friend. Do not engage unless

absolutely necessary. It's the kind of day where agreeing with everything is your best option. Keep a low profile, offer tea, and wait it out.

Thunderstorms
Oh boy, here we go. You're going to need every ounce of patience you've got. Break out the chocolate, offer a massage, or just nod your head in silent agreement. She's in no mood for backtalk, so keep it brief.

Total Meltdown
Sound the alarm and find shelter! Today's a minefield, and one wrong move means you're in the doghouse. Bring out the big guns: her favorite treats, fluffy blankets, and maybe even a peace offering in the form of wine. Brace yourself and don't take anything personally. You'll be lucky if you make it out alive.

Outburst Probability Meter
Think you can predict the likelihood of an outburst today? Rate it on a scale from 1 to 10:
1-3: Unlikely. Might even be a peaceful day.
4-6: Possible. Keep an eye out for triggers.
7-8: Highly Likely. Tread carefully, you're on thin ice.
9-10: Inevitable. Just do yourself a favor and stay out of her way.

Survival Strategies
Depending on today's forecast, follow one of these strategies to improve your chances of survival:

Sunny: Plan an outing, cook her favorite meal, or suggest a movie night. Use this time wisely and soak up the calm.

Partly Cloudy: Stick to safe topics. Compliment her, be agreeable, and stay alert for any change in mood.

Overcast: Lay low. Offer tea, give her space, and try not to attract attention. She'll appreciate your silent support.

Thunderstorms: Apologize in advance for everything. Keep your responses short and sweet, and for the love of sanity, don't argue.

Total Meltdown: Bring out the big treats, keep the compliments coming, and remember: this too shall pass.

Protective Gear for the Day
Keep these essentials handy:

Earplugs: For sudden outbursts.

Noise Canceling Headphones: When you just need to zone out and survive.

Fan: For her hot flashes, and maybe for you when things get intense.

Emergency Treat Stash: Keep her favorite snacks within reach and offer them as peace offerings when the moment calls.

Quick Tips:
- Be prepared for any emotional "weather"—mood swings can be like unpredictable storms.
- Keep an eye on subtle changes in tone and body language to gauge the forecast.

Survival Pro Tips:
Adapt to the mood changes as they come. Flexibility is your best strategy. If the "weather" turns stormy, offer a comforting gesture or a favorite snack.

Last Resort Tips:
In the event of a "downpour," stay calm and give her space. Remember, the forecast changes quickly, so don't get too comfortable with the current mood.

End-of-Day Reflection
Was your forecast spot on or way off the mark? Rate your accuracy here, and jot down any takeaways. The scale:

Nailed It: I'm a mood-swing whisperer.

Close Enough: Missed a few cues, but survived.

Total Disaster: Misread everything. Spent half the day hiding.

Hot Flash Readiness Kit

Introduction
Alright, here's the cold, hard truth: she's about to go from zero to hellfire in 10 seconds flat. We're talking heat waves that make the Sahara feel like a damn day spa. If you're not prepared, you'll be sweating bullets right along with her. So, consider this your official Hot Flash Readiness Kit. It's got the tools to cool her down before she turns the living room into a furnace and you into a puddle.

Pro tip: keep a fan handy, have ice packs in every freezer nook, and for the love of all things holy, don't ever, EVER, say, "Are you sure it's that hot?" unless you want to sleep outside. Let's keep you frostier than an igloo.

Cooling Essentials Checklist
Mini Fan: Stars for effectiveness, from feels like a breeze to total lifesaver.

Ice Packs: Write down where you've stashed them for quick access.

Cold Treats: Keep a stash of popsicles or frozen grapes ready for offering.

Cooling Towel or Gel Pads: Keep one nearby at all times. It's not just a life-saver; it's a life preserver.

Emergency Response Guide
Mild Warmth: Hand her a cool drink and a mini fan. Act

casual, like it's no big deal.

It's Getting Hot: Offer an ice pack, turn on the fan, and resist any urge to comment.

Molten Lava: Deploy all cooling items at once, open every window, and be prepared for anything.

Absolute Inferno: Hand her the whole damn freezer if you have to. This is not the time to joke.

Flashback Moments
Record any especially memorable hot flashes and what you learned, like, "Always have a cold towel ready," or "Never mention the thermostat."

Cooling Effectiveness Tracker
Rate each item's cooling power:
Mini Fan: Did it save the day?
Cold Water: From barely helped to miracle cure.
Ice Pack: How many seconds of relief did it bring

Quick Tips:
- Keep fans and ice packs on standby for emergency cooldowns.
- Have a cold drink ready to offer without her needing to ask.

Survival Pro Tips:
- Avoid making comments about her temperature. Just help her cool down.
- Stay out of the way, but be close enough to assist if she

needs you.

Last Resort Tips:
- If it gets too intense, suggest a relaxing activity in a cool spot.
- Remember, she's dealing with internal heat, so show empathy.

Mood Swing Bingo

Introduction
Welcome to the game of your life - literally. This isn't your regular bingo; this is Mood Swing Bingo, where you track her highs, lows, and WTF moments, all while scoring points for surviving each one. Think of it as a way to stay sane and maybe even have a laugh (quietly, though).

Here's how it works: every time you spot a classic mood swing, mark it off your card. Five in a row? BINGO, baby! Treat yourself to a victory beer, because you've earned it.

The Bingo Card
Every time you experience one of these classic menopause moments, mark it down. Once you get five in a row, you win... well, mostly your own respect.

Random Crying: Tears appear out of nowhere. Just nod, offer a tissue, and avoid asking, "What's wrong?" unless you want to prolong it.

Sudden Rage: You're walking on eggshells one minute, and the next, she's a volcano. Take cover and remember, don't engage.

Unprovoked Laugh Attack: Out of the blue, something sends her into hysterics. You might not get it, but enjoy the calm while it lasts.

Silent Treatment: She's barely said a word for hours, and you're not even sure what you did. Tiptoe around until she breaks the silence.

Temperature Change: She was hot a minute ago, and now she's shivering. Adjust the thermostat and don't make any snide comments.

Mood Swing Within 2 Minutes: You saw it happen - a total 180 on the mood scale in less time than it takes to microwave popcorn.

Chocolate Demand: She asks for chocolate with the kind of urgency usually reserved for natural disasters.

Serious Organization Frenzy: She's sorting, cleaning, or rearranging like her life depends on it. Best not to get in the way.

Extra Sass: Her sarcasm is next-level today. Smile, nod, and don't try to match it.

How to Play
Mark off each mood as you encounter it. When you complete a row, treat yourself:

Snack Reward: Grab a beer, enjoy a snack, or claim TV remote rights.

Mental Reward: Five minutes of peace and quiet—if you can find it.

Bragging Rights: Quietly celebrate your survival skills.
Bonus Round

Mood Swing Encore: When you get the same mood swing twice in a row, mark it with a star. You can exchange two stars for an extra "get out of jail free" card (i.e.permission to run errands solo).

Quick Tips:
- Prepare for a range of emotions—each day could be different.
- Listen more than you speak. Respond with understanding.

Survival Pro Tips:
- Don't react immediately; give her mood time to settle.
- Know that these changes are part of the process—don't take them personally.

Last Resort Tips:
- If things escalate, remain calm and be supportive without trying to "fix" anything.
- Keep a steady supply of snacks and drinks on hand to help smooth over difficult moments.

Snack Pacification Handbook

Introduction
Here's a pro tip: when things get heated, snacks can be your best friend (and hers too). The right treat at the right time can save you from a lot of grief. This section is all about using food as a peace offering, a distraction, or a way to show you care without saying a word. Think of it as edible diplomacy, when in doubt, bring snacks.

Snack Hierarchy
Match the snack to the mood. Choose wisely, and don't skimp on quality if you know what's good for you.

Mild Grumpiness: Offer her a piece of chocolate or some chips. It's not an emergency, but a little boost won't hurt.

Moderate Irritation: Bring out the big guns, like nachos or a cheese platter. Something with a little extra effort can go a long way.

Full-Blown Rage: She's in DEFCON 1. Go all out with her absolute favorite treat—a pint of ice cream, fancy chocolates, or maybe even her favorite meal delivered ASAP.

Bribery Strategy
Think of snacks as peace offerings. Here's how to present them without making things worse:

Nonchalant Approach: "Hey, thought you might want a

snack." Place it within reach and back away slowly.

Apology Add-On: "Sorry if I've been a pain today. Here's a little something to make up for it." (Works best with chocolate or wine.)

Emergency Tactic: If she's on the verge of a meltdown, hand her the treat with no words. Just deliver and retreat.

Snack Stash Ideas
You'll need to stay stocked up. Here's where to keep emergency treats for easy access:

Glove Compartment: Keep a stash of granola bars or chocolate for car rides.

Nightstand Drawer: Have some dried fruit or cookies on standby.

Office Desk: Sneak some snacks there too - you never know when a quick "I found these for you" moment will come in handy.

Snack Effectiveness Tracker
After each snack mission, rate its success on a scale of 1 to 5 stars:
1 Star: She barely noticed. Maybe even rolled her eyes.
2 Stars: Mildly helped, but didn't change the mood.
3 Stars: Definitely perked her up.
4 Stars: She smiled and thanked you. A rare success!
5 Stars: Instant calm. You're now officially a snack ninja.

Restock Reminders

Use this space to write down any particular treats she loved or requested. The more prepared you are, the better chance you have of staying out of the line of fire.

Quick Tips:
- Snacks are crucial. Replenish the supply often and keep it fully stocked.
- Prioritize her favorite treats and keep them readily available.

Survival Pro Tips:
- Hide a backup stash just in case you run low.
- Have a variety of sweet, salty, and healthy options on hand.

Last Resort Tips:
- In an emergency, prioritize chocolate first—other snacks can follow.
- Remember, a well-timed snack offering can diffuse tension.

Man Cave Escape Plan

Introduction
Some days, the best way to survive is to just get the hell out of the way. You're going to need a solid escape plan for those moments when tensions are high, and silence is golden. Consider this your tactical guide to building the ultimate man cave retreat because sometimes "disappearing" for a while is the only thing that'll keep you sane.

Hideout Ranking
Plan your hideout spots with these ratings in mind:

Garage: Reliable, out of sight, and with enough space for a comfy chair and maybe even a beer fridge.
Rating: High Comfort, Low Detection Risk.

Basement: Decent option if you've got a cozy setup down there. Wi-Fi is a must if you're planning to stay a while.
Rating: Moderate Comfort, Moderate Detection Risk.

Shed: Top-tier option for those in need of real solitude. Bring a jacket and some snacks—it's worth it.
Rating: Medium Comfort, Low Detection Risk.

Bathroom: Short-term hideout only. Believable excuse, but don't push your luck by staying too long.
Rating: Low Comfort, Low Detection Risk (if timed well).

Escape Excuse Tracker

Not every excuse will cut it. Keep a list of reliable ones here, and rate their effectiveness:

"I need to check on the car."
Effectiveness: 8/10. Believable and potentially time consuming if you play it right.

"I'm taking out the trash."
Effectiveness: 6/10. Short escape window, but great for a quick reset.

"Heading to the hardware store."
Effectiveness: 10/10. This is the Holy Grail of excuses. Nobody questions the hardware store. Take your time.

Stash and Supplies Checklist

Your hideouts need the essentials. Use this checklist to stock up:

Snacks: Protein bars, chips, or something non-perishable. You don't want to run out mid-hideout.

Blanket: If you're stuck in the garage or shed, this will keep you warm and comfy.

Charged Phone: In case she needs to reach you. Or, you know, for YouTube.

Reading Material: A magazine, book, or even this survival guide to remind yourself why you're here.

New Hideout Ideas

In case your usual spots get discovered, jot down some new potential retreats.

Neighbor's Garage: Maybe he'll even have a better setup than yours.

Local Café: Wi-Fi, coffee, and absolutely zero chance of running into a meltdown.

Parked Car: When you need some quiet time but can't leave the house, just sit in the car and enjoy the silence.

Quick Tips:
- Designate a space that's all yours for those moments when you need to retreat.
- Stock your man cave with essentials—snacks, comfortable seating, and entertainment.

Survival Pro Tips:
- Keep a stash of emergency supplies here: chocolate (for her or you), your favorite drinks, and maybe a good book.
- Have items that help you relax, like a small fan, a cozy blanket, or headphones for music.

Last Resort Tips:
- If the day has been intense, retreat to your man cave to recharge before re-engaging.
- Your man cave is your sanctuary, so treat it as a peaceful escape where you can regroup and return with renewed patience.

The Pillow Fort Refuge

Introduction
Sometimes, a simple man cave isn't enough. You're going to need a Pillow Fort Refuge - a cozy, peaceful retreat where you can ride out any storm in comfort. Not only will it keep you hidden, but it can also double as a peace offering zone. Build it right, and you might even tempt her to join you in there for some much needed calm.

Here's how to set up your fortress of solitude

Building Instructions
Think of this as constructing your own fortress of sanity. Grab your essentials, and follow these steps:

Gather Your Pillows: The more, the better. Don't hold back.

Blankets: Layer them on thick for ultimate comfort. Soft and fluffy is the way to go.

Soft Lighting: String up some fairy lights if you're feeling fancy. No bright lights allowed.

Music and Earbuds: Create a playlist of calming tunes. If you're sharing the fort, stick to ambient music.

Snacks and Beverages: A stash of treats, water, and maybe even a little "fort wine" if things get tense.

Supply Checklist

Your Pillow Fort needs some essentials. Use this checklist to make sure you're fully stocked:

Comfy Blanket: The softer, the better.

Extra Pillows: You can never have too many. Go for plush if you can.

Portable Speaker: Soft music goes a long way.

Snacks: Pick stuff that doesn't crunch too loud, keep it fort-friendly.

Calm Scents: If you're into candles, lavender or eucalyptus can do wonders. Just make sure it's not flammable.

Fort Names

Let's make this official. Name your fort and let her know that it's a safe, quiet place (for both of you). Here are some suggestions:

Menopause Bunker: When things get intense, hide here.

The Chill Zone: Self-explanatory.

Rage Refuge: A gentle reminder that this is a no yelling zone.

Calm Castle: Because inside here, all is peaceful.

Pillow Fort Rules

Now that your fort is built, you need ground rules. Here's what you and any visitors (like her) need to agree to:

No Talking Unless Necessary: Silence is golden in the fort.

Bring a Snack to Enter: It's an offering of peace.

Leave Your Stress Outside: This is a tension-free zone. Only Soft Music Allowed: If it's louder than a whisper, it's banned.

Respect the Fort: Take care of this sacred space—it might just save your sanity.

Pillow Fort Playlist

Suggestions for your fortress soundtrack:

Calming Instrumentals: Nature sounds, lo-fi, or chill vibes only.

Classics: Whatever feels comforting and quiet.
White Noise: When in doubt, rain sounds or ocean waves can work wonders.

Your Own Choices: Fill in some of your own picks below:

Quick Tips:
- Set up a makeshift pillow fort with plenty of blankets and soft pillows for a comforting hideaway.
- Keep it simple, this refuge is about creating a cozy space to unwind and recharge.

Survival Pro Tips:
- Stock your pillow fort with essentials like snacks, a book, and a soft throw blanket.
- Use the fort for quiet time, whether it's for reading, a nap, or just a peaceful retreat from the day.

Last-Resort Tips:
- If things get overwhelming, retreat to your fort and take some deep breaths. It's your personal escape.
- Bring a small fan or a warm drink, depending on the season, to make it even more comfortable. This is your sanctuary, so enjoy it!

The Menopause First Aid Kit

Introduction
We're in crisis mode here, and no crisis is complete without a fully-stocked first aid kit. This isn't just any kit; it's specifically designed for menopause emergencies. Think of it as your go to stash for soothing, calming, and surviving whatever the day throws at you. Let's make sure you've got everything you need to tackle the heat waves, mood swings, and whatever else menopause decides to dish out.

Essential Items
Make sure you've got these on hand, ready to go at a moment's notice:

Cooling Mist Spray: A quick spritz might just be the difference between sanity and a meltdown. Store it in the fridge for maximum effect.

Lavender Oil: A few drops can calm things down. Dab some on her wrist or diffuse it nearby, but don't get too heavy-handed.

Soft Socks: This might seem basic, but comfy socks are a small luxury that can make a big difference on a rough day.

Heating Pad: Useful for when the chills come after the hot flashes. Also great for any aches or pains she might be dealing with.

Favorite Tea Bags: Chamomile, peppermint, or any other

soothing blend she enjoys. If things get really intense, have some strong chamomile ready.

Relaxation Tools

These extras can go a long way in helping her chill out (and you too).

Massage Ball: Great for when tension hits hard. Roll it over her shoulders, or just offer it to her with a "go on, treat yourself" look.

Eye Mask: Perfect for shutting out the world and taking a breather. You might even want to get a matching one so you can join her for a nap.

Headphones: For her calming music or your personal noise-canceling sanctuary. Either way, headphones are a must.

Weighted Blanket: The hug you both need when life's a little too much. If you don't already have one, consider it an investment in your survival.

Comfort Station Setup

Designate a cozy corner in the house as a comfort station and keep it stocked:

Pillows and Blankets: Soft, cozy, and inviting. A place she can escape to when the world gets too loud.

Calming Scents: Essential oils or candles with eucalyptus, lavender, or chamomile.

Entertainment: A stack of her favorite books or a loaded Kindle. Maybe add a note that says, "If you need anything, don't hesitate to ask, but no rush."

Quick-Fix Recipes
Emergency relaxation on the fly. Try these quick fixes when things are on the verge:

Chamomile Tea: Boil water, steep tea, and serve with a slice of lemon if you're feeling fancy.

Epsom Salt Foot Soak: Fill a tub with warm water, add Epsom salts, and offer it to her as a mini spa moment. She'll appreciate it, and you'll get a few minutes of quiet.

Herbal Compress: Heat a damp washcloth with a few drops of lavender oil in the microwave for 10-15 seconds. Apply to her neck or shoulders for instant relaxation.

Your Personal First Aid Kit
You'll need some essentials, too. Stock up on:
Earplugs: In case things get too intense.

Noise-Canceling Headphones: For when you need a solo escape.

Energy Drink: To keep up with the pace of survival mode.

An Extra Beer: For after things have cooled down, and you've made it through another day.

Quick Tips:
- Keep this kit fully stocked and within easy reach, you'll want it ready at a moment's notice.
- Include basic essentials like a mini fan, chocolate, and a comforting tea.

Survival Pro Tips:
- Tailor the kit to her needs: add items like cooling towels, lavender oil, and maybe a little notebook for tracking what works best.
- Restock frequently. Items like chocolate and her favorite snacks should never run out.

Last Resort Tips:
- Use the kit as your go-to in any crisis—hand her an item without hesitation, whether it's chocolate, a cool cloth, or a comforting drink.
- Keep emergency extras hidden in various places around the house, like the car or your man cave, so you're always prepared. This kit is your lifeline, so treat it as such!

Menopause Proof Conversation Guide

Introduction
When it comes to conversations, you're going to need to tread carefully. Menopause isn't just hot flashes and mood swings; it's also a minefield of potential conversational traps. Lucky for you, this guide is here to help you navigate these tricky waters with a list of things you can (and should never) say, along with some foolproof phrases to help you stay on her good side.

Phrases to Use
These are your conversational life-savers. When in doubt, stick to these and you'll minimize the risk of setting her off:

"I'm listening."
You'd be surprised how far these two words will get you. Say it sincerely and with a nod.

"That sounds frustrating."
Simple, supportive, and you don't need to have any idea what she's actually talking about.

"I'm here for you."
Solidarity. Reassurance. You're telling her she's not alone in this, and that matters.

"How can I help?"
This one's gold. Offer it up without any expectation of a specific answer, and be prepared for anything.

Phrases to Avoid

Don't even think about saying these unless you're actively seeking trouble:

"Calm down."
Just… don't. You might as well set off a flare in a field of dry grass.

"Is it really that bad?"
Yes, it is. And asking her this will only make it worse.

"Are you sure it's menopause?"
This is not the time to question her experience. If she says it's menopause, it's menopause.

"You're overreacting."
Congratulations, you just volunteered for the next decade on the couch.

Apology Templates

When you inevitably screw up, here are some ready made apologies to fall back on. Fill in the blanks, and remember to sound sincere:

"I'm sorry I didn't realize ___. I know now that ___, and next time, I'll ___."

Use this for any offense, big or small. It's like the Swiss Army knife of apologies.

"I didn't mean to ___, and I'm sorry if it made you feel ___. I'll do better."
Acknowledge her feelings, apologize, and promise to improve. Solid move.

"You're right, I wasn't thinking. How can I make it up to you?"
You're basically surrendering, and that's okay. This one shows humility and a willingness to get it right next time.
Compliment Generator

Here's your secret weapon.
When all else fails, a well-timed compliment can work wonders. Try these on for size:

"You're handling this with such strength."
Points for acknowledging her toughness.

"You look fantastic today."
Even if she knows it's cheesy, she'll appreciate the effort.

"I'm really proud of you."
She's dealing with a lot, and hearing this will mean something.

Reassurance Toolkit
Write down a few specific things she likes to hear and keep them on hand for when you need an extra dose of charm. Here are some to get you started:

"You're amazing."
"Thank you for everything you do."

"I couldn't do this without you."

Feel free to personalize these and use them generously. Sometimes, a little reassurance is all it takes to turn a day around.

Quick Tips:
- Stick to light and positive topics whenever possible—think happy memories, shared interests, or future plans.
- Avoid potentially sensitive subjects like the thermostat, sleep, or anything involving change.

Survival Pro Tips:
- Listen more than you talk. Show you're engaged by nodding and responding thoughtfully.
- Have a few go-to questions ready that are neutral and reassuring, like "How was your day?" or "What would make you feel relaxed right now?"

Last Resort Tips:
- If the conversation starts to feel tense, gently steer it toward something fun or calming.
- Remember, you don't have to solve her problems, sometimes she just needs to vent. Offer empathy and a listening ear, and keep your responses positive.

The Eye Roll Counter

Introduction
If you've made it this far, then you're no stranger to "the look." You know the one - a classic, slow-motion eye roll that lets you know exactly how much you've screwed up, without a single word. Consider this your Eye Roll Counter, a place to keep track of every side eye, sarcastic squint, and over the top roll she throws your way. With a little practice, you'll become an expert in spotting the warning signs and (maybe) avoiding a few in the future.

The Daily Eye-Roll Tracker
For each eye roll you encounter, record the details here. Over time, you'll build a handy catalog of "what not to do" moments.

Eye Roll #1
What You Said or Did: _____
Severity Scale:
Mild (1): Barely noticeable. She's annoyed but not too upset.
Moderate (5): A classic roll. You're on thin ice.
Severe (10): Full head tilt and maybe even a sigh. You've really done it now.
Reaction Outcome: Circle one:
Ignored You
Gave You "The Look"
Added Sarcasm for Good Measure

Eye Roll #2
What You Said or Did: _____

Severity Scale: (Same 1-10 scale as above)
Reaction Outcome: Circle one:
Silent Treatment Initiated
Left the Room
Told You Exactly What You Did Wrong

Eye Roll Severity Scale
Let's break it down. Use this scale to rate each eye-roll, because, yes, they come in levels:

1-3: She's mildly annoyed. You could probably redeem yourself with a joke. Proceed cautiously.

4-6: Solid eye-roll territory. Backpedal if you can, and try a quick compliment.

7-8: This is where things get serious. Apologize now or face the consequences.

9-10: Full-blown rage-roll. You might need to bring out the big guns: chocolate, tea, or total silence.

Weekly Recap
At the end of the week, tally up your eye rolls and reflect on any trends. Are certain topics triggering the roll? Are you saying something consistently that's pushing her buttons? Write it down here and consider it a warning sign for next week.

Quick Tips:
- Don't take the eye roll personally, it's often more about the

situation than about you.
- Respond with a gentle smile or a knowing nod, showing you're taking it in stride.

Survival Pro Tips:
- Avoid making things worse by asking "What's wrong?" right after an eye roll. Give it a moment to pass.
- If you sense another eye roll coming, pause and reconsider your words. Sometimes silence is the safest response.

Last Resort Tips:
- Treat the eye roll as a warning sign, and steer the conversation to safer ground.
- If you're feeling bold, respond with a lighthearted comment like, "Ah, the classic eye roll, I know that one well." Just make sure the timing is right!

Chill Level Tracker

Introduction
You know what they say: "Happy wife, happy life." Well, in the world of menopause, you're going to need more than just happiness - you need to monitor her "chill factor." The Chill Level Tracker lets you rate her calmness (or lack thereof) throughout the day. This way, you can adapt, survive, and possibly even thrive by knowing when to push your luck and when to keep your head down.

Daily Chill Levels
Track her "chill" throughout the day in three stages: Morning, Afternoon, and Night. This gives you a full day's read on her mood shifts and helps you navigate the safest path.

Morning Chill
Rating:
Zen (1): You're in the clear. Start the day with light conversation and keep things positive.

Neutral (5): No major signs of irritation, but stay alert.

Gale Force Winds (10): It's going to be a bumpy ride. Lay low and hope for the best.

Best Approach: _____

Afternoon Chill
Rating: (Use same 1-10 scale as above)
Best Approach: _____

Night Chill
Rating: (Use same 1-10 scale as above)
Best Approach: _____

Mood Triggers to Watch For
Log any major mood shifts or triggers you spot. This is where you'll take note of the things that affect her "chill" the most.

Common triggers might include:
Housework Unfinished: If you promised to do something and didn't, brace yourself.

Temperature Change: Rapidly changing weather can sometimes bring on the "heat."

Random Noise: Loud TV? Barking dog? Silence might be your safest bet.

Use this space to add her unique mood triggers:

Chill Level Survival Tips
Depending on the chill level, here's how to best handle each situation:

1-3 (Zen): Engage, enjoy, and make her laugh. These days are gold.

4-6 (Neutral): Keep it simple and pleasant. Avoid stirring the pot.

7-8 (Edgy): Tiptoe. Stick to agreeable topics, and be ready to switch gears if her mood dips.

9-10 (Stormy): You're in survival mode. Respond minimally, stay out of the way, and avoid all sarcasm.

End-of-Day Chill Reflection
Summarize today's chill level in one sentence: _____
_____

Add any notes for future reference, especially if you found a successful tactic:

Quick Tips:
- Keep an eye on the overall vibe. If things feel tense, take proactive steps to help her relax.
- Stay aware of her chill level throughout the day—notice if she seems unusually quiet, tense, or irritable.

Survival Pro Tips:
- Have a few calming strategies ready to go, like suggesting

a soothing activity, offering her favorite drink, or simply giving her space.
- Make a habit of checking in with her mood without being intrusive. A simple "How's it going?" can help gauge the chill level.

Last Resort Tips:
- If the chill level drops significantly, bring out the "big guns": chocolate, her favorite show, or a cozy blanket.

- Remember, staying calm yourself can help improve the overall chill level. Lead by example, and keep things as relaxed as possible.

Sage Advice You Wish You Hadn't Given

Introduction
Sometimes you just can't help yourself. You're trying to be helpful, and before you know it, you've offered a nugget of advice that seemed brilliant in your head - but she definitely didn't want to hear it. This section is where you document those moments of Sage Advice You Wish You Hadn't Given. It's a chance to learn from your mistakes, so maybe next time, you'll think twice before speaking up.

Daily Advice Log
For each instance, record the following details to build a catalog of "what not to say" moments:

Today's Unwanted Advice
What You Said: _____

Her Reaction:
Mildly Annoyed: Eye-roll, slight sigh, but no lasting damage.

Shut Down: She gave you the silent treatment, maybe even left the room.

Triggered a Rant: Yep, you hit a nerve. Be prepared for a long lecture.

Outcome:
Ignored Completely
Politely Dismissed

Escalated Quickly

Notes for Next Time: _____

Common Offenses
Here are some repeat offenders that tend to go down like a lead balloon. Check them off when you've made the mistake and add new ones as needed:

"Have you tried just relaxing?"
Oh, so she just needs to relax? Good one. Maybe next, you can suggest breathing exercises.

"Maybe you're overthinking it."
Congratulations, you just implied she's too emotional. Be prepared for a counterattack.

"Are you sure it's that bad?"
Rookie move. Never question the severity. If she says it's bad, it's bad. End of story.

Reflection Section
At the end of each week, reflect on any particularly bad advice moments. Use this space to make a mental note for future conversations:

What Worked: If something surprisingly didn't backfire, record it here.

What Bombed: Highlight the biggest flops of the week.
Next Time, Try Saying…: Write down alternative phrases you can use instead, like "I can only imagine" or "That must be tough."

Alternative Suggestions
Fill in a few go-to responses that you can fall back on when you're tempted to give advice. This way, you'll be ready with something neutral, yet supportive:

"I'm here if you need me."
"That sounds rough. How can I help?"
"I can see why you'd feel that way."

Quick Tips:
- Avoid offering advice unless she explicitly asks for it, sometimes listening is all she needs.
- When in doubt, keep your suggestions to yourself, and focus on being supportive instead.

Survival Pro Tips:
- If you feel compelled to share advice, frame it as a personal observation ("What works for me is…"), rather than direct guidance.

- Offer validation first: "I totally understand why you feel that way." Then, gauge her response before saying anything else.

Last Resort Tips:
- If you've already offered advice and it didn't go over well, apologize and shift back to listening.
- Remember, she may not be looking for solutions—just someone who listens without judgment. Keep the advice to a minimum, and save yourself the trouble!

The Apology Bingo

Introduction
Welcome to Apology Bingo! You're going to be saying "I'm sorry" a lot during this time, so why not make a game out of it? Apology Bingo lets you track all the different ways you've had to apologize this week. Get five in a row, and you've earned yourself a treat. Hey, if you're going to mess up anyway, you might as well make it fun.

The Bingo Card
Each time you find yourself apologizing, mark it off on the bingo card below. When you've completed a row, reward yourself with a snack, a drink, or a bit of peace and quiet.

Apologized for No Reason: You're not sure why, but it seemed safer to just say sorry.

Said Sorry and It Wasn't Enough: Apology accepted? Nope. She's still not happy.

Admitted You Were Wrong (Again): Sometimes it's easier to just take the blame.
She Was Right. You realized it, admitted it, and said sorry. Classic.

Agreed Just to End It: You apologized just to get out of an argument. Smart move.

Big-Time Screw-Up: This was a serious apology. Extra points if you had to grovel.

Repeated the Apology: Turns out, once wasn't enough.

In the Doghouse: This apology might not even be enough to fix things.

Bought Her a Peace Offering: You combined the apology with chocolate, wine, or something shiny.

How to Play
Mark each square as you go along. Five in a row, column, or diagonal? BINGO! Reward yourself with one of the following: Snack Reward: Indulge in some beer, a treat, or maybe just a few minutes of silence.

Get Out of Jail Free: If you score two bingos in one week, you get a free pass to escape for a while.

Bonus Reward: If you manage to fill the entire card, take yourself out for a long walk, a solo coffee run, or whatever brings you joy (and peace).

End-of-Week Apology Recap
Look back at the bingos you scored this week and reflect on any particular trends:

Apology MVP: Did any one apology dominate the board? Write it here.

Biggest Lesson Learned: Jot down anything you learned from this week's apologies.

Next Week's Goal: Set a target, like "Try not to apologize for things that aren't my fault" (good luck with that).

Emergency Apology Kit
Fill this space with your go-to apologies for any occasion:

The Classic: "I'm sorry, I didn't mean to upset you."

The All-Inclusive: "I'm sorry for whatever I did, whatever I might do, and whatever you think I'm planning to do."

The Sincere: "I'm really sorry I didn't think, and I should have. I'll do better next time."

If you're running low on fresh apologies, don't worry, repeating one from earlier in the week is totally acceptable. The trick is to sound sincere, even if you're on your fifth apology of the day.

Quick Tips:
- Sincere, quick apologies work best. Don't overthink it —just apologize and move forward.
- Keep your apologies simple and direct. Sometimes, "I'm

sorry" is all you need to say.

Survival Pro Tips:
- Have a list of go-to apologies ready for different situations, like "I didn't mean that" or "I'll do better next time."
- Pair an apology with a small gesture, like offering her favorite treat or making a comforting cup of tea.

Last Resort Tips:
- If you've used the same apology too often, switch it up to keep it fresh: "That's on me—I'm really sorry."
- Avoid justifying your actions immediately after apologizing. Give her space to respond before explaining.

The Side Eye Diary

Introduction
Ah, the side-eye. Subtle, yet deadly. You'll be getting this look a lot during menopause, it's the universal sign that you've said something dumb, done something wrong, or just exist in her space at the wrong moment. Consider this your Side Eye Diary, a place to log each "Really?" glare, along with a few notes on what earned you that honor. Learn from these moments, and maybe, just maybe you'll avoid a few down the road.

The Side Eye Log
For each side eye moment, document the details so you'll remember what to steer clear of in the future.

Side Eye #1
What You Did: _____

Severity Scale:
Mild (1): Barely noticeable. She was annoyed but let it slide.

Medium (5): Full-on glare. She wants you to know you're on thin ice.

Severe (10). The mother of all side eyes. She's ready to roast you.

Outcome:
Sigh
Silence
Sarcastic Comment

Notes for Next Time: _____

Side-Eye #2
What You Did: _____
Severity Scale: (Use the same 1-10 scale as above)

Outcome:
She Left the Room
Rolled Her Eyes So Hard It Hurt
Gave You the Cold Shoulder
Notes for Next Time: _____

Severity Breakdown
Side eyes aren't created equal. Here's a quick guide to decode them:

1-3: The "I don't have time to deal with this" side eye. Safe to say, you can apologize and move on.

4-6: The "Are you really that clueless?" side eye. You've probably annoyed her - might be best to lay low.

7-8: The "Seriously?" side eye. Tread carefully; you're walking on eggshells now.

9-10: The "I am this close to losing it" side eye. You've officially pissed her off. Apologize, bring peace offerings, and proceed with extreme caution.

End of Week Side Eye Recap
Take a moment to reflect on the week's side eyes and any

recurring themes:

Most Common Offense: Record the things that keep landing you in side eye territory.

Takeaway Lesson: Jot down what you've learned, if anything.

Avoid Next Week: Write down any habits you plan to change, like "No more jokes about the thermostat."

Quick Tips:
- Recognize the side eye as a silent cue, it often means you should stop, listen, or reconsider your last move.
- Respond with a gentle nod or a knowing smile to acknowledge the look without escalating.

Survival Pro Tips:
- Treat the side-eye as a feedback mechanism. Take it as a hint to change course or adjust your approach.
- If you're on the receiving end, a quiet "Noted" or "I see what you're saying" can help defuse tension.

Last Resort Tips:
- The side eye is a signal to tread carefully. Avoid reacting defensively, and instead shift into listening mode.
- If it becomes a frequent occurrence, make mental notes of what triggers it and adjust accordingly. Consider it an opportunity to refine your survival strategy!

The Temperature of the Room

Introduction
You're about to become intimately familiar with the phrase "hot and cold." She'll be freezing one minute and sweating the next. Here's your Temperature of the Room tracker, a guide to help you survive the rapid shifts in her internal thermostat without losing your mind. This section will help you log her hot flashes, chilly moments, and the immediate actions you took to keep the peace.

Temperature Tracker
Monitor the room's temperature and your responses at different times of the day. Use this as your guide to know when to adjust the thermostat, bring out the fan, or just back away slowly.

Morning Temperature
Temperature Rating:
Freezing (1): She's bundled up and complaining it's like the Arctic. Blanket time.

Chilly (5): Just cold enough that you might need to close a window or hand her some tea.

Blazing (10): She's ready to rip the windows open, crank the fans, or both.
Your Action Taken: _____

Afternoon Temperature
Temperature Rating: (Same 1-10 scale as above)

Your Action Taken: _____

Evening Temperature
Temperature Rating: (Same 1-10 scale as above)
Your Action Taken: _____

Temperature-Based Actions
Depending on the room's temperature, here's your cheat sheet for how to respond:

1-3 (Freezing): Hand over a cozy blanket, heat up a mug of tea, and avoid any comments about the temperature.

4-6 (Chilly): A sweater or hoodie should do the trick. Offer one with zero sarcasm.

7-8 (Warm): Get ready to hear complaints about the heat. Crack a window or, if she doesn't want the AC, just agree with whatever she says.

9-10 (Blazing): Bring out the fan, offer ice water, and step back. She's in the danger zone, and you do not want to mess with this level of heat.

Cooling Supplies Checklist
Keep these handy, because you never know when you'll need them:
Fans: Mini, hand held, or full blown standing fan, keep a variety at the ready.

Ice Packs: The cooler, the better. Have them stashed in the freezer for quick deployment.

Cool Washcloths: Toss one in the freezer for those emergency situations.

Frozen Treats: Keep popsicles or frozen grapes on hand to offer as "cooling gifts."

End-of-Day Temperature Reflection
Use this space to reflect on how well you handled today's temperature shifts:

What Worked: Anything that helped cool things down or warm things up successfully.

What to Avoid: Actions or comments that made things worse. Maybe today's the day you learned not to mention the thermostat at all.

Next Time: Any tips for your future self, like "Pre-freeze the ice packs" or "Keep blankets in plain sight."

Quick Tips:

- Respect her temperature preferences. The thermostat is sacred ground.
- Don't adjust it without her knowledge unless absolutely necessary.

Survival Pro Tips:

- Invest in extra blankets or layers for yourself if the temperature feels too cool.
- Make adjustments quietly and subtly to avoid detection.

Last Resort Tips:

If you're caught, play it off as a technical check.

Remember, maintaining her comfort is the ultimate goal.

Chocolate Bribery Log

Introduction
When in doubt, chocolate. This isn't just a snack; it's a tool for peace, a bridge over troubled waters, and sometimes the only thing standing between you and a meltdown (hers or yours). Welcome to the Chocolate Bribery Log, where you'll keep track of every sweet offering you've made in the name of harmony. You'll want to note what worked, what bombed, and how much chocolate you should probably keep stocked from now on.

Daily Bribery Log
For each bribe attempt, record the details so you'll know what to reach for in the future. Trust me, this will come in handy.

Bribery Attempt #1
Type of Chocolate: _____

Presentation Style:
Casual Drop-Off: "Oh, I found this for you."

Peace Offering: "I thought you could use a little treat."

Desperate Attempt: "Please don't kill me. Here, take it."

Effectiveness Rating:
1 Star: She barely noticed. Might need to upgrade to something fancier.

3 Stars: Mildly improved the mood. Not bad for an emergency.

5 Stars: Instant success. She's happy, you're safe, all is right with the world.

Notes for Next Time: _____

Bribery Attempt #2
Type of Chocolate: _____

Presentation Style: (Use the same choices as above)

Effectiveness Rating: (Use the same 1-5 star scale)

Notes for Next Time: _____

Bribery Strategies
Here's your quick guide on how to deliver chocolate like a pro:

Nonchalant Approach: Casually leave the chocolate on her desk, the counter, or wherever she'll see it. No grand gesture necessary, sometimes, subtlety is key.

The Full Presentation: Bring it to her with a beverage of choice (tea, wine, coffee). Add a note like, "You deserve this" for bonus points.

Emergency Tactic: If the mood is especially stormy, hand over the chocolate with no words. Just a silent, supportive gesture. This says "I get it" without saying anything at all.

Top Bribery Choices
Stock up on these crowd pleasers. You never know when you'll need them:

Fancy Chocolates: Think of the good stuff—nothing less than 70% cocoa. You're looking to impress.

Dark Chocolate Bars: A classic. Simple, but effective.

Chocolate Covered Anything: Strawberries, nuts, pretzels, if it's covered in chocolate, it's a win.

Truffles: Because sometimes, only the best will do.

Restock Alert
Use this space to note any favorites so you'll remember to grab extras:

Weekly Bribery Recap
At the end of each week, reflect on what worked best and what to adjust:

Most Effective Chocolate: _____

Biggest Bribery Fail: _____

Next Week's Plan: Stock up on more of what worked and steer clear of anything that didn't cut it.

Quick Tips:
- Always have a stash of chocolate on hand, don't wait until it runs out.
- Know her favorite types and brands by heart.

Survival Pro Tips:
- Keep an emergency backup hidden, just in case.
- Restock regularly to ensure there's always fresh chocolate available.

Last Resort Tips:
- If you're out, make a quick trip to replenish the supply. No delays.
- Chocolate is more than a treat; it's a crucial part of your survival toolkit.

Moods to Dodge Today

Introduction
Some days, the best way to survive is to avoid certain topics and situations altogether. This is where Moods to Dodge Today comes in handy. Use this section to track potential mood triggers and dodge them like a pro. After all, sometimes it's less about fixing the mood and more about staying out of its way.

Today's Top Moods to Avoid
These are the red flags. If any of these apply, proceed with caution:

Easily Irritated: Little things are setting her off. Avoid any unnecessary questions, and for the love of all things holy, do NOT comment on her tone.

Silent but Deadly: She's not saying much, but you can feel the tension. Approach with extreme caution. This is not the time to ask, "What's wrong?"

Melancholy Movie Time: She's got a sad movie on, and the tears are coming. Sit quietly, offer tissues, and don't try to "fix" anything.

Organizing Spree: She's in full rearrange-the-closets mode. Keep out of the way, and for God's sake, don't suggest a different method.

How to Spot Today's Triggers

Look for signs early in the day so you can plan your moves:

Temperature Shifts: If she's fluctuating between hot and cold, it might be best to just agree with everything and move on.

Room Changes: If she's pacing between rooms or obsessing over a project, stay out of her way and let her be. Now's not the time for small talk.

Housework Focus: If she's hyper focused on chores, grab a broom and look busy, or simply disappear. You do not want to be seen lounging when she's in this mood.

Avoidance Strategy Guide

When in doubt, here's how to navigate today's touchy moods:

For Easily Irritated: Stay neutral. No jokes, no sarcasm, no commentary. Keep a straight face and agree with everything.

For Silent but Deadly: Do not ask questions. Sometimes, saying less is the best way to dodge a storm.

For Melancholy Movie Time: Sit with her, offer comfort, but keep your opinions to yourself. If she cries, hand over tissues silently and be supportive.

For Organizing Spree: Be "helpful" but not intrusive. Or, better yet, just steer clear of her path altogether.

Escape Plan of the Day

Once you've identified today's mood triggers, use this space to outline an escape plan. Example strategies:

Offer to Run Errands: Need anything from the store? Now's a great time to volunteer.

Suggest a Movie Night: Something she likes that's soothing and distracting.

Retreat to the Man Cave: If she's in organizing mode, let her have the house to herself and get to the man cave stat.

End-of-Day Reflection

Rate how well you dodged the moods today:

1 (Barely Made It): Today was rough. You're lucky you survived.

5 (Ninja Level Dodging): You avoided every trap and emerged unscathed. Victory!

Takeaway Lesson: Write down what you learned, and use it as future survival knowledge.

Quick Tips:
- Pay attention to subtle cues and adjust your approach based on her mood. If she seems tense, be extra mindful.
- If you sense a challenging mood, keep interactions light and focus on offering support, not solutions.

Survival Pro Tips:

- Prepare for unpredictable shifts by having a few comforting gestures ready, like a warm drink, a snack, or a soothing playlist.
- Avoid controversial topics, and stick to safe, positive subjects to keep things calm.

Last Resort Tips:

If things feel particularly tense, step back and give her some space. Often, a bit of breathing room helps defuse the mood. Recognize that some days call for extra patience. Stay calm, go with the flow, and remember that you'll get through it together.

The "Can I Help?" Gauge

Introduction
Ah, the classic question: "Can I help?" It seems like a simple enough offer, but depending on the mood, it can be either a hero move or a fast track to trouble. The "Can I Help?" Gauge will guide you through knowing when to ask, what to offer, and when to just leave well enough alone. Because sometimes the best way to help is to simply stay out of the way.

The Daily Help-O-Meter
Assess the situation before you offer to help. Rate the likelihood of your offer being well-received, based on the mood you're walking into:

Level 1 (Hero's Welcome): She's in a decent mood and will probably appreciate the help. This is a green light to offer, and she might even thank you for it.

Level 5 (Proceed with Caution): There's a 50/50 chance. You can offer, but be prepared for her to either accept with conditions or turn you down outright. Tread lightly.

Level 10 (Danger Zone): Abort mission. You'll probably make things worse by offering to help. Today is a day to stay quiet, look busy, and avoid getting in her way.

Today's Offer Log
For each attempt, jot down what you offered and how it went. You'll soon get a feel for what's safe and what's risky.

Attempt #1
What You Offered: _____

Response:
Grateful: She appreciated the offer and let you help.

Mildly Annoyed: You could tell she was on the fence but let you help anyway.

Turned You Down: She insisted on doing it herself. Take the hint.

Result:
Success: You helped without issue.
Neutral: No harm, no foul.
Regret: She declined with a side of sarcasm. Best to stay away for a bit.

Notes for Future Reference: _____

Attempt #2
What You Offered: _____

Response: (Use the same choices as above)

Result: (Use the same options as above)

Notes for Future Reference: _____

When to Offer Help

Use these pointers to help you decide when an offer will go over well:

Safe Times to Offer:
When she's actively doing something and seems slightly overwhelmed.

When she's visibly annoyed by something specific (and you know how to fix it).

If she directly sighs or looks around as if she could use a hand.

Bad Times to Offer:
When she's quiet but clearly deep in thought. Do not disturb.

When she's visibly tense, hot, or in the middle of a hot flash.

Offering to help now might seem like you're saying she can't handle it.

During moments of organization. It's her territory now, don't trespass.

Future "Help" Suggestions

Jot down things you can safely offer to help with, based on past successes:
Offer to Do the Dishes: If she hates this chore, you might score some points.

Take Over Dinner Plans: Food can be a welcome distraction, especially if she doesn't have to cook it.

Handle the Laundry: A small gesture, but sometimes it's the little things.

Reflection on Today's Help Attempts
Use this space to reflect on how your offers were received, and any lessons for next time:
Biggest Win: _____
_____

Lesson Learned: _____
_____

Next Time, I'll Offer…: Write down any plans for future helpful gestures.

Quick Tips:
- Only ask "Can I help?" if you're ready to follow through.
- If you sense she needs support, offer it with no strings attached.
- Phrase your offer thoughtfully, like "Would you like a hand with that?" or "Is there anything you'd prefer I handle?"

Survival Pro Tips:
- Observe before offering help, sometimes just being present is enough. If she seems frustrated, offer a specific way you can assist.
- Be prepared for her to decline. If she does, respect her choice and stay supportive in other ways.

Last Resort Tips:
- If she seems annoyed by your offer, gently back off and say, "I'm here if you change your mind."
- Sometimes she may just need a listening ear rather than direct help. Keep your focus on her needs, and be ready to adjust accordingly.

End of the Day Debrief

Introduction
Congratulations, you survived another day! The End of the Day Debrief is where you get to reflect on what you did right, where you went wrong, and what you'll do differently tomorrow. Consider this a daily pat on the back (or kick in the pants) for how you handled the mood swings, hot flashes, and side eyes. It's your chance to track any small wins, big lessons, and essential takeaways.

Today's High Point
What went well today? Record any moments of success, big or small, that made it feel like you weren't just running for cover:

Today's Low Point
Alright, what bombed? Did you say something stupid, miss a cue, or otherwise step in it? Use this space to reflect on your worst moment of the day:

Survival Tip Learned Today
Each day brings its own set of lessons. Write down anything you learned that you think might help you tomorrow. Remember, you're building up your survival skills here:

Tomorrow's Game Plan
Based on today's experiences, outline a strategy for tomorrow. This can be as simple as "Keep quiet until noon" or as specific as "Start the day with coffee and chocolate in hand." Whatever works:

Overall Survival Rating
Rate your performance today on a scale from "Nailed It" to "Needs Improvement":

Nailed It: I kept my cool, dodged the mood swings, and got a smile or two.

Close Enough: Missed a few cues but survived.

Total Disaster: Misread everything and spent half the day hiding.

Use this scale to give yourself a daily grade. Hey, nobody's perfect, but you're giving it a shot.

Quick Tips:
- Recap the day to yourself, noting what worked and what didn't.
- Give yourself credit for handling it all, no matter how it went.

Survival Pro Tips:
- Reflect on ways to improve and keep doing what works well.
- Stay patient, progress is about learning and adjusting.

Last Resort Tips:

Remind yourself that each day is a chance to try again. Self-compassion goes a long way. You're doing your best!

The "Keep Your Mouth Shut" Game

Introduction
Some days, the best move you can make is keeping your mouth shut. It sounds simple, but trust me, it's a skill. In The "Keep Your Mouth Shut" Game, you'll face scenarios that seem like great opportunities to offer advice, crack a joke, or make a comment - until you realize you've just opened the door to trouble. In this game, you'll learn to recognize when to bite your tongue, nod along, and stay silent. Ready to give it a try?

Game Rules
For each scenario, you'll have a few response options. Choose the one you'd normally go for, and then check the rating to see if you'd survive. Hint: the right answer is usually the one where you say the least. Let's play.

Scenario 1: She's Complaining About the Heat
She's fanning herself, muttering about how hot it is, and glaring at the thermostat. You:

A. Suggest opening a window.
Rating: 2/10. Now you've triggered a debate about fresh air vs. A/C. Just nod and sympathize.

B. Offer to bring her a glass of ice water.
Rating: 8/10. Good move. You're offering help without telling her what to do. You get points for effort.

C. Say, "I don't think it's that hot."

Rating: 0/10. Oh, you've done it now. Prepare for a lecture on how you have no idea what she's going through. Run.

D. Keep your mouth shut and hand her the remote for the A/C.
Rating: 10/10. Silent, supportive, and smart. This is a winning choice.

Scenario 2: She's Cleaning Furiously and Looks Frustrated
The house is spotless, but she's going at it like she's trying to scrub through to the basement. You:

A. Ask, "Isn't the house already clean?"
Rating: 1/10. You've made a rookie mistake. Do not question her cleaning logic. You're about to get an earful.

B. Offer to help and ask what needs to be done.
Rating: 9/10. Nice one. She might even hand you a duster and appreciate the support.

C. Make a joke about "cleaning rage."
Rating: 3/10. You thought you were being funny, but now you're just adding fuel to the fire.

D. Keep your mouth shut and quietly start vacuuming.
Rating: 10/10. Silent support without commentary. She'll appreciate the effort (or at least leave you alone).

Scenario 3. She's Having a Meltdown Over Something Small. You're not entirely sure what set her off, but she's visibly upset and venting. You:

A. Tell her to calm down.
Rating: 0/10. Huge mistake. Never in the history of arguments has this gone well.

B. Nod and say, "I'm here for you."
Rating: 10/10. Perfect response. No need for extra words, just show you're present and supportive.

C. Try to fix the problem for her.
Rating: 4/10. Your intentions are good, but now she feels patronized. Back off.

D. Listen, keep your mouth shut, and hand her a tissue.
Rating: 9/10. A solid choice. You're showing support without interrupting. Well done.

Scorecard
30 Points or More: You're a pro at keeping quiet. Enjoy the peace and maybe treat yourself to a reward.

20-29 Points: Pretty good, but there's room for improvement. Remember, less is often more.

19 Points or Fewer: You've got some work to do. When in doubt, stay silent and just nod along.

Quick Tips:
- Some situations call for silence, less is more.
- If she's speaking, avoid interjecting unless invited.

Survival Pro Tips:
- Observe her cues and gauge if she wants a response or just a listening ear.
- Only respond when it feels safe to do so. Choose your words carefully.

Last Resort Tips:
- If you feel unsure, saying nothing is usually better than risking the wrong thing.
- Keep nodding, and let her vent if she needs to, it's therapeutic for both of you.

The Menopausal Mood Dictionary

Introduction
Welcome to The Menopausal Mood Dictionary, your quick reference guide to decoding the range of moods you'll encounter. This isn't just a dictionary; it's a survival tool, complete with explanations and tips for handling each mood. Whether she's in full meltdown mode or suspiciously calm, this section will help you understand what's going on and what you should (or shouldn't) do about it.

Mood: The Hot Flash Frenzy
Description: She's uncomfortably hot and radiating heat like a small sun. You can practically see the steam coming off her.

How to Spot It: She's flushed, fanning herself, and might be peeling off layers faster than you can blink.

Survival Tips:
- Offer an ice pack or a glass of cold water.
- Open windows or hand her the fan without comment.
- DO NOT, under any circumstances, mention the thermostat
- or make any jokes about her internal temperature.

Mood: The Silent Treatment
Description: She's gone radio silent, and you're not entirely sure why. You're left in the dark, trying to piece together what went wrong.

How to Spot It: She's giving short answers or ignoring you completely. There's an aura of quiet intensity.

Survival Tips:
- Don't ask, "What's wrong?" Instead, try offering tea or a snack.
- Give her space, but check in occasionally with gentle gestures.
- Use this time to reflect on your recent comments and think of an apology, just in case.

Mood: The Cryfest
Description: She's crying over something that might seem small or random. It could be a commercial, a song, or just life in general.

How to Spot It: The tears are rolling, and she's sniffling. It's possible she's clutching a tissue.

Survival Tips:
- Hand her tissues without asking questions. Let her vent, and listen.
- Offer a comforting statement like, "I'm here for you."
- Do NOT try to fix the problem. Just be present.

Mood: The Organizing Frenzy
Description: She's in full reorganization mode, tackling closets, drawers, and cabinets like she's on a mission.

How to Spot It: She's got cleaning supplies in hand, and you can hear the sound of drawers being pulled open and slammed shut.

Survival Tips:
- Stay out of her way. If you want to help, ask gently if she needs anything.
- Avoid making comments about the mess or asking why she's organizing.
- If possible, pitch in with a small task, but be prepared to retreat if she prefers to work solo.

Mood: The Burst of Energy
Description: Suddenly, she's got all the energy in the world and is tackling projects left and right. You're not sure where it came from, but you're along for the ride.

How to Spot It: She's moving quickly, talking faster, and taking on projects. It's almost like she's had five espressos.

Survival Tips:
- Go with the flow. If she asks for help, be ready to jump in.
- Don't question her motivation or try to slow her down.
- Offer encouragement and stay positive. She's on a roll, and you're just here to support.

Additional Moods to Watch For
Use this space to add any unique moods you encounter:

Quick Tips:
- Take note of her mood and adjust your approach accordingly, tuning into the emotional "language" of the day can make all the difference.
- When in doubt, offer quiet support. Sometimes simply acknowledging her mood with a smile or a nod is enough.

Survival Pro Tips:
- Use her mood as a guide for the day's interactions. If she's feeling low, suggest a comforting activity; if she's upbeat, join in and enjoy the moment.
- Keep a few mood-boosters on standby: chocolate, a warm drink, a light-hearted movie suggestion. Adapt to the mood with flexibility.

Last Resort Tips:
If the mood shifts rapidly, go with the flow - don't question it. Respond with calm reassurance, and avoid taking anything personally.
Remember, moods are often temporary. Stay patient, and show that you're there for her no matter what the day brings.

Top 10 Things You Should Never, Ever Say

Introduction
Consider this your survival bible, the Top 10 Things You Should Never, Ever Say. These phrases are the equivalent of jumping into a shark tank with a steak around your neck. If you value your sanity (and your life), read them, memorize them, and then pretend you've never even thought of them. Avoid these statements at all costs, and you'll dodge at least 90% of potential disaster. Ready? Let's get into the top 10 phrases that will take you straight from "oh no" to "hell no."

The Top 10 "Do Not Say" Phrases

"Calm down."
Why It's a Disaster: Might as well have said, "Keep going, please, get even madder." This one's the ultimate mood grenade. If you ever find this phrase rolling off your tongue, bite it, hard, and back away slowly.

"Are you sure it's menopause?"
Why It's a Disaster: Oh, you're questioning her? Bold move. This isn't an episode of House MD, and you're not her doctor. If she says it's menopause, it's menopause. If she says it's a space alien invasion, it's that too. Just go with it.

"It can't be that bad."
Why It's a Disaster: You're saying this to the woman who's experiencing 300-degree hot flashes and mood swings that could make a rollercoaster look stable. Next time, try: "That sounds intense. How can I help?" and watch the magic

happen.

"You're overreacting."
Why It's a Disaster: Ah, the classic. Telling someone they're overreacting usually leads to, you guessed it, an even bigger reaction. It's like handing her a megaphone and asking her to go louder. Go silent, and avoid eye contact.

"Is it that time of the month?"
Why It's a Disaster: Have a seat. This is not a menstruation issue, and suggesting it is a ticket to Couch City for the next week. If you value your evenings, skip this one. Forever.

"Why are you so emotional?"
Why It's a Disaster: Imagine someone told you this right after you stubbed your toe on the coffee table for the third time. This line is like putting a match to dry leaves, it's a fast and explosive mistake. She doesn't need analysis; she needs chocolate.

"I liked it better when…"
Why It's a Disaster: You're waxing nostalgic about the past? Dangerous territory, buddy. Stick to "I love how things are now" and be done with it. Safer that way.

"I don't think it's that hot in here."
Why It's a Disaster: You're questioning her experience of a hot flash? Brave, but foolish. It's hot in here, because she said so. Hand her a fan, offer an ice pack, and step away. Repeat as needed.

"Do you really need more chocolate?"
Why It's a Disaster: If there was ever a question you should not ask, it's this one. She needs all the chocolate she can get, and she needs it now. Asking this is like denying a firefighter water. Just keep the stash stocked and pass it over with a smile.

"Maybe you just need to exercise more."
Why It's a Disaster: Oh, you've done it now. She wasn't looking for a personal trainer. The next words out of your mouth should be, "How about a spa day?" and nothing else. Trust me on this one.

Bonus "Don't You Dare"
If you find yourself reaching for any variation of "Are you feeling better now?" stop, drop, and roll right out of the room. This phrase can only go one way, and it's downhill. Fast. Instead, try this timeless classic: silence. Sometimes, not speaking is the best thing you can do for both of you.

Takeaway
These phrases are the equivalent of poking a bear with a stick. Avoid them at all costs. And if you can't remember them all, just remember this: if it sounds like advice, sounds like a critique, or even remotely sounds like you know better, skip it. Grab her a cup of tea, nod supportively, and keep your mouth shut.

Quick Tips:
- Think twice before speaking, if it sounds risky, it probably is! Stick to safe topics and steer clear of anything that might

provoke.
- Avoid phrases that suggest she's overreacting, like "Calm down" or "It's not that bad." These are guaranteed to backfire.

Survival Pro Tips:
- Replace potentially problematic phrases with neutral ones. For instance, instead of saying, "Are you sure it's menopause?" try, "I'm here to help however you need."
- Keep a mental list of phrases to avoid, like anything that questions her feelings, her age, or her temperature control choices.

Last Resort Tips:
- If you slip up and say one of the forbidden phrases, apologize immediately and pivot to something comforting.
- Remember, some topics are best left alone. If in doubt, stay quiet, smile, and let her lead the conversation.

Weekly Survival Scorecard

Introduction
Congratulations, you made it through another week! This Weekly Survival Scorecard is your chance to reflect on your ups, downs, and the genius strategies that kept you alive. Think of it as your personal scoreboard for navigating the menopause obstacle course. The goal here is simple: celebrate your wins, learn from your losses, and prepare to do it all over again next week. Ready to tally up the damage?

Weekly Survival Highlights
Fill in your best moments, because you've earned a little self-praise:

Top Win of the Week: What did you absolutely crush this week? Whether it was biting your tongue at the right moment, delivering the perfect snack, or just not messing up for a change, note it here.

Most Impressive Escape: When did you make a flawless getaway? Write down that time you dodged a potential blow-up like a pro.

Biggest Save: The snack, apology, or offer that truly saved the day. Remember this one for future use.

Weekly Survival Stats
Rate yourself in these critical areas and see where you stand on the survival spectrum:

Bingo Achievements: How many rows did you complete on Apology Bingo? _____ rows

Side-Eyes Dodged: Estimate the number of side-eyes you successfully avoided. _____ side-eyes

Moods Dodged: How many days did you spot the moods early and steer clear? _____ days

Chocolate Deployments: Total times you used chocolate as a peace offering. _____ times

Weekly Reflection
Take a moment to reflect on what you learned, and maybe, where you could have done better:

What Worked: This week, what strategy actually made life easier? Whether it was silence, snacks, or strategic exits, record it here.

What Backfired: Let's face it, something probably went wrong. What was your biggest regret this week?

Survival Tip for Next Week: Based on this week's wins and losses, what's one thing you'll do differently?

Overall Survival Rating
Give yourself a rating on a scale from "Nailed It" to "Should've Stayed in Bed":

Nailed It: You're practically a menopause whisperer. Enjoy a well-deserved beer.

Pretty Good: Made it through with minimal damage, and learned a thing or two.

Barely Survived: You scraped by, but it wasn't pretty. Maybe next week, try the "Keep Your Mouth Shut" game a little harder.

Should've Stayed in Bed: We've all had those weeks. Try to forget it, restock the chocolate, and get ready for a fresh start.

Quick Tips:
- At the end of each week, take a few minutes to reflect on your survival skills, celebrate your wins and note what could

improve.
- Rate your week based on how well you handled key situations. Did you avoid major pitfalls? Did you successfully use humor and empathy?

Survival Pro Tips:
- Use the scorecard to track your best tactics and strategies.
- If something worked well, repeat it next week!
- Give yourself bonus points for moments of patience, well-timed compliments, and successful snack diplomacy.

Last Resort Tips:
If the week was tough, focus on the positive moments and make a plan for small adjustments moving forward. Remember, surviving another week with humor and grace is an achievement in itself. Reward yourself for making it through and approach the new week with fresh resolve.

Future Planning: The Survival Kit Restock Guide

Introduction
You've made it through a week or two, and now you're starting to realize that survival requires supplies. This Survival Kit Restock Guide will help you keep your kit fully stocked and ready for anything. Think of it as a checklist of essentials to get you through the next meltdown, hot flash, or mood swing. Because let's be honest: running out of chocolate mid-crisis is not an option. Take a deep breath, grab a pen, and let's make sure you're ready for the next round.

The Essentials
Use this list as your guide for weekly restocks. Check it off as you go, because you never know when you'll need each item:

Chocolate
Restock Level: Minimum of one box, ideally a variety pack. Think dark, milk, truffles, and maybe some chocolate covered almonds.
Preferred Brands: _____

Cooling Gear
Restock Level: Fresh ice packs (swap out the old ones), a functional mini fan, and maybe an extra cooling towel.
Recommended Quantity: At least one per room, just in case.

Special Note: Don't forget to rotate these back to the freezer after each use.

Soothing Beverages
Restock Level: Enough chamomile tea for at least a month and a couple of bottles of her favorite wine.
Extra Options: Herbal teas, calming blends, or even some nice sparkling water for non-wine nights.

Emergency Snacks
Restock Level: Assorted snacks that she loves. Stock up on nuts, crackers, cheese, or anything else that's quick and satisfying.
Secret Stash Spots: Consider keeping these in a few hidden locations for last minute peace offerings.

Comfort Kit Refill
Here are the must-haves to keep her feeling cozy and pampered:
Soft Socks and Blankets: Make sure you have fresh, fluffy socks in her favorite colors and a couple of new blankets if the old ones are looking worn.
Cozy Blankets: Check for soft textures, weighted options, or even an electric blanket if she likes extra warmth.

Aromatherapy Supplies:
Restock Level: Fresh lavender oil, eucalyptus, or chamomile. Replace any candles you've burned through, and check the diffusers to make sure they're good to go.

Bonus: Restock the Apology Kit

If you find yourself repeating apologies too often, it's time to expand your repertoire. Jot down any new go-to lines here that worked well over the past week:

New Apology Phrases:

Additions to the "Silent Gesture" Collection:

A quick shoulder rub, a warm mug of tea, or a fresh snack on standby. Add anything that proved effective here.

Your Future Plan

Once you've restocked, think ahead. What new items could make the next week easier? Use this space to jot down any ideas:

Possible Additions:

With this guide, you'll be fully prepared for whatever menopause throws at you. Restock regularly, stay sharp, and remember: when in doubt, chocolate is always the answer.

Quick Tips:
- Schedule a regular restock of your survival essentials, like chocolate, calming tea, and extra batteries for the fan. Make it a habit to check your kit weekly.
- Keep a checklist of items that are running low, so you're never caught unprepared in a moment of need.

Survival Pro Tips:
- Consider keeping duplicates of high use items (like chocolate) in multiple spots around the house, just in case.
- Review your kit every month to see if there's anything new you could add based on recent experiences. Adaptability is key!

Last Resort Tips:
- If supplies run low, prioritize items that make the biggest difference, like her favorite snacks and quick mood-boosters.
- Remember, a well-stocked survival kit is essential for maintaining peace and staying ready for whatever comes your way. Preparation is your best strategy!

25 Menopause Survival Multiple Choice Quiz

1. If She's Giving You "The Look," You Should:
A. Smile and ask, "What's wrong?"
Bold move. But you're basically asking for a meltdown.

B. Apologize immediately, even if you don't know what for.
This is a solid strategy. Preemptive apologies are like Kevlar in this situation.

C. Pretend you didn't see it and quietly start doing the dishes.
Ah, the old "silent chore defense." Smart. She can't yell if you're being helpful... hopefully.

2. What's the Most Essential Item in Your Menopause Survival Kit?
A. A Fire Extinguisher
For those hot flashes that could practically ignite furniture.

B. Earplugs and a Pillow
Perfect for when you need a quick escape to the couch (or to hide under it).

C. A Library of Apologies
Why stop at one apology when you can have an arsenal? This way, you're ready for any situation.

3. When She Sighs and Rolls Her Eyes, She's Really Saying:
A. "Please, by all means, keep talking."

Oh no, no. This means exactly the opposite. Move to silence immediately.

B. "I'm giving you a second chance to backtrack and correct whatever you just said."
A sigh is like a warning shot. Do NOT ignore it.

C. "It's time to get out the chocolate and stop asking questions."
Now you're getting it. A peace offering might be your only hope at this point.

4. The Safest Response to "Does This Make Me Look Fat?" Is:
A. "No, you look amazing!"
A classic, but tread carefully. Be sincere, or risk detection.

B. "Maybe a different color would be more flattering?"
Congratulations, you've chosen the express route to the doghouse. Grab a pillow.

C. "How about we skip this question and go get some ice cream?"
Distraction through snacks! It's a bold strategy, but sometimes a tactical retreat is best.

5. Which of the Following Is NOT a Safe Topic of Conversation During Menopause?
A. The Thermostat Settings
Talking about the thermostat is like tossing a match into a dry forest—nothing good can come of it.

B. Her New Favorite Show
This one's relatively safe, as long as you remember all the characters and their backstories.

C. Plans for a Quiet Night In
Almost always a good choice—especially if it involves chocolate and silence.

6. When She Says "I'm Fine," What Does She Really Mean?
A. "Everything is okay. Let's move on."
Sorry, friend. She might say she's fine, but this is a universal code for "You'd better fix whatever you just broke."

B. "I need you to figure out what's wrong and fix it, now."
This is the correct interpretation. Time to break out the survival kit and get to work.

C. "I'm so happy with you right now."
You're dreaming. This answer does not exist in the real world.

7. If You're Caught Off Guard by a Mood Swing, Your Best Course of Action Is:
A. Ask her, "Is everything okay?"
Why, oh why, would you choose this? Abort mission and find a new strategy.

B. Hand her a cup of tea, a piece of chocolate, and walk away slowly.
Now we're talking! Leave the scene and let the chocolate do

the heavy lifting.

C. Smile and try to distract her with a joke.
Risky move. A joke could make things better or far, far worse. Proceed with caution.

8. What's the Most Likely Outcome if You Adjust the Thermostat Without Telling Her?
A. She'll immediately notice and lecture you on the importance of respecting her body temperature control.
Yep, she has thermostat radar. You've been warned.

B. She won't notice and thank you later.
If you believe this, you haven't been paying attention. She's going to notice.

C. You'll spend the next hour adjusting it back to exactly where it was.
This is the most likely scenario. You're going to end up right back where you started.

9. When She Asks, "What Are You Thinking About?" Your Safest Response Is:
A. "Nothing."
She'll never believe it. Go with something a little more thoughtful.

B. "How lucky I am to have you."
This one's a classic for a reason. Sure, it's cheesy, but she'll love it.

C. "Wondering how much I can get for my golf clubs."
Bold, but unnecessary. This is not the time for financial musings.

10. The Best Time to Offer a Peace Offering of Chocolate Is:
A. When she seems frustrated with work or life in general.
Good call! Chocolate soothes the soul, and the timing couldn't be better.

B. Right after she's finished telling you what you did wrong.
Even better. Chocolate has a way of softening any critique.

C. Right after you've eaten the last piece in the stash.
This is dangerous territory. She'll notice, and there's no stash big enough to save you from the fallout.

11. You Hear Her Rummaging Through the Cabinets for a Late-Night Snack. You Should:
A. Quietly pretend you didn't hear anything.
Sometimes, stealth is the best policy.

B. Offer to go grab her favorite snack from the store.
Nice move. It's late, but nothing says devotion like a snack run.

C. Yell from the other room, "Are you hungry again?"
Risky. You may end up sleeping in the kitchen tonight.

12. She Decides to Vent About Her Friend Drama. Your Job Is To:
A. Listen attentively and say, "That sounds tough."
Great choice! You're showing empathy without getting tangled in the details.

B. Offer advice on how she should handle it.
She wasn't looking for your opinion. Just listen, and take notes if you have to.

C. Take her friend's side to be "devil's advocate."
Devil's advocate? You just became the devil. Good luck with that.

13. She's in the Middle of a Rant About Something Minor. You Should:
A. Nod, agree, and let her get it all out.
Good call! Sometimes, the best thing you can do is just be a supportive audience.

B. Offer her a glass of wine to take the edge off.
This could work well—just make sure it's her favorite, and don't mention why you're offering.

C. Tell her it's not a big deal and suggest she calm down.
Congratulations, you just opened the door to a full-blown argument. Backpedal now!

14. What's the Best Thing to Do When She's Having a Moment of Self-Doubt?
A. Tell her she's overreacting and needs to toughen up.

Yeah… no. This is not the pep talk she's looking for. Try a different approach.

B. Tell her how amazing she is and list all her strengths.
Nailed it! A good ego boost is exactly what she needs.

C. Walk away and give her space to "deal with it."
She's not going to appreciate that. She's looking for support, not a disappearing act.

15. If She Catches You on Your Phone While She's Talking to You, You Should:
A. Quickly put the phone down and say, "I'm all ears!"
Nice recovery! A little enthusiasm goes a long way.

B. Keep scrolling and hope she didn't notice.
She noticed. She always notices. Prepare for a lecture on paying attention.

C. Explain you were just looking up something she mentioned.
Not bad—she might appreciate the effort. Just make sure you really were, or this won't end well.

16. She's in Full Cleaning Mode and Clearly on a Mission. You Should:
A. Offer to help, but only with the easy stuff.
Good strategy. Show you're willing, but don't get in the way.

B. Hide in the garage until it blows over.
Sometimes a tactical retreat is wise, but if she catches you,

you're done for.

C. Suggest she take a break and relax.
Careful! This could be seen as an insult. Better just jump in and lend a hand.

17. The Correct Response to "Do You Think I've Gained Weight?" Is:

A. "No way! You look exactly the same."
Solid answer. Just make sure to say it with confidence.

B. "Maybe a little, but who hasn't?"
Yikes! She's not looking for honesty—she's looking for reassurance. Choose again.

C. "You look fantastic. I wouldn't change a thing."
Perfect! Safe and reassuring. You're a quick learner.

18. She Asks If You Remember Your Wedding Anniversary. You Should:

A. Rattle off the date and make up a sweet memory on the spot.
A+ for effort! She'll love the sentiment, even if it's a little improvised.

B. Guess and hope you're close enough.
Oof. This could end badly. If you're not sure, don't guess—look it up!

C. Stall and try to change the subject.
Bold strategy, but she's not going to let you off the hook that

easily. Better come prepared.

19. If She's Having a Day Where She Hates Everything, You Should:

A. Try to cheer her up with jokes and a funny story.
Proceed with caution—she might not be in the mood for laughs. But hey, points for effort!

B. Offer to take her out for a treat or her favorite meal.
Great choice! A little indulgence goes a long way, especially on a rough day.

C. Tell her it's just a phase and she'll get over it.
You're looking at a long night on the couch. Never minimize her feelings.

20. You Come Home to Find She's in a Terrible Mood. Your First Move Is:

A. Ask her what's wrong and try to talk it out.
She might appreciate this—or she might just want to stew. Be prepared for either.

B. Hand her a glass of wine and retreat to a safe distance.
Wise choice! Offer support from a distance, and you just might survive.

C. Try to tell her about your own tough day.
This is not the time to one-up her. Put your day on hold and be there for hers.

21. When She Comes Back from Shopping and Asks for Your Opinion on Her New Outfit, You Should:

A. Compliment it like it's the most stunning thing you've ever seen.
Safe move! She wants validation, not a fashion critique.

B. Make a suggestion for a different style that might look better.
Dangerous territory! She didn't ask for a style consultation.

C. Say, "It's nice, but do you really need more clothes?"
RIP. You just signed your own demise. Let's hope you have a comfy couch.

22. She Mentions She's Thinking of Getting a New Haircut. Your Best Response Is:

A. "You'd look amazing no matter what!"
Excellent choice. She's fishing for support, and you're delivering.

B. "Are you sure that's a good idea?"
She was looking for enthusiasm, not doubt. Better keep it positive next time.

C. "Why change it? I like it how it is."
You just implied she's making a mistake. She might be rethinking more than her hair now.

23. She Wants You to Help Out More Around the House. You Should:

A. Immediately start a chore, even if you're not sure what to do.
Showing initiative is a win! She'll appreciate the effort.

B. Tell her you'll do it later when you're less tired.
Later is dangerous territory. She might be less patient than you think.

C. Ask her to make a list of what she wants done.
This can go either way. She might appreciate the clarity, or she might think you're just trying to buy time.

24. She Gets Upset Because You Forgot Something Important. Your Move?

A. Apologize, offer to make it up to her, and actually follow through.
Nailed it! Take responsibility, and don't just promise—deliver.

B. Deflect and try to change the subject.
She's not going to let that fly. Better to face it head-on.

C. Argue that it wasn't actually that important.
Oh no. You just dug yourself into a deeper hole. Start working on an exit strategy.

25. When She Says She Needs Some Space, You Should:

A. Give her space, but let her know you're nearby if she needs you.

Perfect response! You're respecting her wishes while staying supportive.

B. Insist on talking it out, even if she doesn't want to. You're about to experience the true meaning of "needing space." Step back, now.

C. Interpret "space" as an invitation to leave for the weekend. That's a bit too much space. Don't take it personally—just give her the distance she needs.

Daily Survival Prompts - Mini 30 Day Journal

Day 1: Daily Survival Score
Menopausal Mood of the Day
Today, her mood was a mix of: _____ and _____
Emergency Chocolate Count
Chocolate used: _____ Bars | _____ Bites | _____
Reserve Stash
Eye Roll Score
Number of eye rolls I received: _____

Day 2: Tactical Escapes
Best Dodge of the Day
Describe the situation: _____
Top Temperature Debate
Thermostat adjustments made today: _____ | Final setting: _____ °F
Hot Flash Alert Level
How hot was it today? Mild | Steamy | Inferno

Day 3: Chocolate and Compliments
Menopause Proof Compliment of the Day
Compliment I used: _____
Today's Chocolate Resupply Mission
Where I went: _____ |
Did I bring enough? Yes / No
Moment I Earned Husband/Boyfriend Points
What I did: _____ |
Her reaction: _____

Day 4: Most Ridiculous Moments
Most Ridiculous Moment of the Day
Describe it: _____
Sneaky Survival Tactic
Something I did that she didn't notice:

_____

Mood Swing Tracker
Mood swings counted today: _____

Day 5: Reflect & Recover
Today's Best Apology
Apology used: _____
Effectiveness (1-10): _____
Moment of Sweet Relief
When I knew I was safe: _____
Today's Overall Survival Rating
Rate today's experience: _____
Notes: _____

Day 6: Coping Mechanisms
Snack Survival Kit Usage
Snacks used today: Chocolate | Cheese | Wine | Tea
Most Dangerous Phrase I Almost Said
Phrase: _____
How proud am I of my restraint? (1-10): _____
Best Distraction Tactic Used
Describe it: _____
Effectiveness (1-10): _____

Day 7: Emergency Situations
Moment of Triumph
When I got it right today:

_____

Her reaction: _____
Pat on the Back
What did I do well today?

_____

My pride level (1-10): _____
Today's Laugh-Out-Loud Moment
What happened: _____
 Who laughed   _____

Day 8: Mood Management
Mood Swing Tracker
Mood swings counted today: _____
Moment of Zen
One peaceful moment today:

_____

How I felt: _____
Today's Most Surprising Menopause Wisdom
What I learned today: _____

Day 9: Temperature Trouble
Hot Flash Alert Level
Temperature today: Mild | Steamy | Inferno
Moment I Used Chocolate to Diffuse a Situation
Describe the situation: _____
| Did it work? Yes / No
Thermostat Battle Log
Number of adjustments: _____ | Final setting: _____ °F

Day 10: Encouragement and Reflection
Menopause-Proof Compliment of the Day
Compliment I used: _____
Moment I Earned Bonus Points
What I did: _____
Her response _____
Advice I'll Use Tomorrow
Plan for tomorrow: _____

Day 11: Today's Highlights
Today's Chocolate Resupply Mission
Where I went: _____
Did I bring enough? Yes / No
Moment of Sweet Relief
When I knew I was safe for the day:
_____

Top Menopausal Weather Report
Her emotional weather today: Clear Skies | Partly Cloudy | Thunderstorm

Day 12: Humor in the Madness
Funniest Thing I Said That Didn't Get Me in Trouble
Joke or comment: _____
Did she laugh? Yes / No
Best Dodge of the Day
Situation avoided:_____
Sneaky Survival Tactic
Something I did to survive unnoticed:
_____

Day 13: Tracking the Chaos
Most Ridiculous Moment of the Day
Moment: _____
Emergency Chocolate Count
Chocolate used: _____ Bars | _____ Bites | _____
Reserve Stash
Moment I Used Silence as a Survival Tool
Situation: _____
Success level (1-10): _____

Day 14: Apologies and Escapes
Today's Best Apology
Apology used: _____
Effectiveness (1-10): _____
Today's Overall Survival Rating
Rate the experience: _____
Notes: _____
Moment of Sweet Relief
What I did right today: _____

Day 15: Tactical Tricks
Best Distraction Tactic Used
Describe it: _____
Effectiveness (1-10): _____
Words I'll Never Say Again
Phrase to avoid: _____
Today's Mood Control Success
What I did to help maintain the peace:
_____

Day 16: Chocolate and Chill
Emergency Chocolate Count
Chocolate used today: _____ Bars | _____ Bites | _____ Reserve Stash
Moment I Earned Extra Partner Points
What I did: _____
Her reaction: _____
Today's Most Surprising Menopause Wisdom
What I learned: _____

Day 17: Daily Debrief
Most Ridiculous Moment of the Day
Describe it: _____
Mood Swing Tracker
Mood swings counted: _____
My Best Apology Attempt
Apology: _____
Rating (1-10): _____

Day 18: Tactical Moves
Best Dodge of the Day
Describe the situation: _____
Moment of Zen
The peaceful moment today:
_____
Moment I Knew I Was Safe
What I did right: _____

Day 19: Sweet Survival
Snack Survival Kit Usage
Snacks used: Chocolate | Cheese | Wine | Tea
Funniest Thing I Said That Didn't Backfire
Joke or comment: _____
Did she laugh? Yes / No
Today's Chocolate Resupply Mission
Where I went: _____
Did I bring enough? Yes / No

Day 20: Navigating Hot Flashes
Hot Flash Alert Level
Today's heat level: Mild | Steamy | Inferno
Moment of Sweet Relief
Describe the relief moment:
_____

Top Temperature Debate
Thermostat adjustments today: _____ | Final setting: _____ °F

Day 21: A Day in Reflection
Today's Best Compliment
Compliment I used: _____
Pat on the Back
What I did well today: _____
| Pride level (1-10): _____
Moment I Used Silence to Survive
Situation: _____
Success level (1-10): _____

Day 22: Chocolate Diplomacy
Moment I Used Chocolate to Diffuse a Situation
Describe the situation: _____
| Did it work? Yes / No
Today's Best Apology
Apology used: _____
Effectiveness (1-10): _____
Eye Roll Score
How many eye rolls I received: _____

Day 23: The Compliment Arsenal
Menopause-Proof Compliment of the Day
Compliment I used: _____
Her response: _____
Most Dangerous Phrase I Almost Said
Phrase: _____
How proud am I of my restraint? (1-10): _____
Today's Laugh-Out-Loud Moment
What happened: _____
 Who laughed? _____

Day 24: Today's Tactics
Best Distraction Tactic Used
Describe It: _____
Effectiveness (1-10): _____
Sneaky Survival Tactic
Something I did to survive unnoticed:
_____
Advice I'll Use Tomorrow
Plan for tomorrow: _____

Day 25: Reflect and Reward
Moment of Triumph
Describe the win: _____
Her reaction: _____
Moment of Zen
Today's peaceful moment:
_____

Moment I Knew I Was Safe
What I did right today: _____

Day 26: Temperature and Chocolate
Hot Flash Alert Level
Today's heat level: Mild | Steamy | Inferno
Today's Chocolate Resupply Mission
Where I went: _____
Did I bring enough? Yes / No
Thermostat Battle Log
Thermostat adjustments today: _____ | Final setting: _____ °F

Day 27: Emergency Snacks and Mood Control
Snack Survival Kit Usage
Snacks used: Chocolate | Cheese | Wine | Tea
Mood Swing Tracker
Mood swings counted: _____
Moment of Sweet Relief
Describe it: _____

Day 28: Chocolate Diplomacy 2.0
Emergency Chocolate Count
Chocolate used today: _____ Bars | _____ Bites | _____
Reserve Stash
Today's Best Compliment
Compliment I used: _____
Her response: _____
Most Ridiculous Moment of the Day
Describe the moment: _____

Day 29: Humor and Survival
Funniest Thing I Said That Didn't Get Me in Trouble
Joke or comment: _____
Did she laugh? Yes / No
Moment I Earned Extra Partner Points
What I did: _____
Her reaction: _____
Best Dodge of the Day
Describe the situation avoided: _____

Day 30: Today's Wins and Lessons
Today's Overall Survival Rating
Rate today: _____ |
Notes: _____
Pat on the Back
What I did well: _____
Pride level (1-10): _____
Words I'll Never Say Again
Phrase to avoid: _____

Congrats, You Survived!

Well, look at you - you made it to the end! You've tackled mood swings, hot flashes, and the world's most unpredictable thermostat settings. You've sharpened your survival skills, stocked up on chocolate, and probably learned a thing or two about keeping your mouth shut. Most importantly, you've embraced the golden rule of menopause survival: if in doubt, don't ask questions and bring snacks.

The Menopause Survival Checklist: A Final Review
Let's take one last look at your essential survival skills. By now, you should be:

A Chocolate Ninja: Armed with peace offerings at all times. When in doubt, chocolate it out.

A Thermostat Whisperer: You know when to adjust and when to stay far, far away from the temperature controls.

A Master of Silence: You've learned when to smile, nod, and keep your brilliant insights to yourself. You might just be an undercover genius.

A Professional Apologizer: At this point, "I'm sorry" practically rolls off the tongue, and that's a skill worth celebrating.

A Hot Flash First Responder: You know the drill—fan, ice pack, back away slowly. You're practically a pro.

Your Certificate of Survival

Consider yourself officially certified in Menopause Survival. You've earned the right to brag (silently, of course) and perhaps treat yourself to a snack or two - just don't eat the last piece of chocolate without checking with her first.

What's Next?

The journey doesn't end here, my friend. You've got plenty of days ahead filled with weather forecasts, chocolate deliveries, and the occasional game of "guess what I did wrong." But you're ready for it. With this guide in hand, you'll not only survive - you'll thrive. Because let's be honest, you're now practically an expert on the art of "yes, dear" and the fine balance of keeping her happy while keeping your sanity.

Final Words of Wisdom

Remember, menopause isn't a phase. It's a lifestyle. So go forth with confidence, courage, and a fully stocked survival kit. And if all else fails, remember the golden rule: when in doubt, just say yes and hand over the snacks.

So here's to you - the ultimate Menopause Survivor. You've earned every laugh, every eye roll dodge, and every quiet night on the couch. Now go grab yourself a celebratory drink. You've earned it.

The End (Or the Beginning of the Rest of Your Survival Skills).